The Magic of Microgreens
Book Two – Radish

By
Errol Williams

Occam's Publishing
P.O. Box 333
Palm Harbor, Fl 34682

THE MAGIC OF MICROGREENS – Radish
Book Two
Copyright © 2024 by Errol Williams

An Occam book.
Published by Occam's Publishing
P.O. Box 333
Palm Harbor, Fl 34682

Williams, Errol
    The Magic of Microgreens / Errol Williams
Book Two - Radish

First Edition: September 2024

Printed In the United States Of America

0 9 8 7 6 5 4 3 2 1

Chapter 1: Introduction to Radish Microgreens

Understanding Microgreens

Understanding microgreens opens a world of possibilities for health-conscious individuals eager to enhance their diets and embrace sustainable practices. Microgreens are young, edible plants harvested just after the first true leaves develop, offering a concentrated source of nutrients. Among these vibrant greens, radish microgreens stand out for their robust flavor and impressive health benefits. They are not only easy to grow but also add a delightful crunch and peppery taste to various dishes, making them a favorite among culinary enthusiasts.

The nutritional profile of radish microgreens is remarkably rich, packed with vitamins, minerals, and antioxidants that support overall health and wellness. Studies have shown that they can contain up to 40 times more nutrients than their mature counterparts. This makes them an excellent addition to any diet, especially for those looking to boost their intake of essential nutrients without consuming large quantities of food. Including radish microgreens in your meals can help improve digestion, support immune function, and provide a wealth of anti-inflammatory benefits, promoting a healthier lifestyle.

Urban farming has gained significant momentum, and radish microgreens are perfect for city dwellers with limited space. Their compact growth habit allows them to thrive in small containers or even hydroponic systems, making them accessible for anyone interested in cultivating their own food. This not only fosters a deeper connection to the food we eat but also empowers individuals to take charge of their nutrition. Furthermore, growing microgreens at home ensures that you have fresh, organic produce at your fingertips, reducing reliance on store-bought options that may lack quality and freshness.

Pest management is an essential aspect of cultivating radish microgreens, especially for those who prioritize organic methods. By implementing sustainable practices, such as companion planting and natural pest deterrents, growers can minimize the need for chemical interventions. This approach not only protects the health of the plants but also contributes to a healthier environment. Embracing these eco-friendly strategies ensures that your microgreens are grown in a manner that aligns with your health-conscious values while maintaining the integrity of the produce.

Finally, the culinary versatility of radish microgreens makes them an exciting ingredient to experiment with in the kitchen. They can be used as a garnish, added to salads, blended into smoothies, or incorporated into sandwiches and wraps. Their vibrant color and distinct flavor enhance both the aesthetic and taste of dishes, encouraging individuals to explore new culinary creations. By integrating radish microgreens into your meals, you not only elevate your dining experience but also nourish your body with the incredible benefits these tiny greens offer. Embrace the journey of understanding microgreens, and let them transform your approach to health and wellness.

The Unique Qualities of Radish Microgreens

Radish microgreens stand out not only for their vibrant colors but also for their impressive nutritional profile. Packed with vitamins A, C, E, and K, these tiny greens offer a concentrated dose of essential nutrients in a small package. The high levels of antioxidants present in radish microgreens help combat oxidative stress, making them a fantastic addition to a health-conscious diet. With their low calorie count and high fiber content, they are ideal for anyone seeking to enhance their meals without compromising on nutrition.

One unique quality of radish microgreens is their remarkable flavor profile. They possess a peppery, slightly spicy taste that can elevate a dish from ordinary to extraordinary. Whether tossed in salads, blended into smoothies, or used as a garnish, they add a delightful kick to various culinary creations. This versatility makes them a favorite among chefs and home cooks alike, providing an easy way to enhance flavor while boosting nutritional value. Incorporating radish microgreens into your meals not only supports your health but also enriches your culinary experience.

In addition to their culinary advantages, radish microgreens are incredibly easy to grow, making them perfect for urban farming initiatives. They thrive in small spaces, requiring minimal equipment and resources. With just a few seed trays and some soil, anyone can start cultivating these greens right in their kitchen or balcony. This accessibility empowers individuals to take charge of their food sources, promoting self-sufficiency and sustainable practices. Urban farming with radish microgreens also helps reduce the carbon footprint associated with transporting produce, making it an environmentally friendly choice.

Pest management is another area where radish microgreens shine. Their rapid growth cycle means they can be harvested quickly, reducing the time for pests to establish themselves. Additionally, their natural peppery flavor can deter certain pests, minimizing the need for chemical interventions. For those committed to organic farming practices, this quality allows for a healthier growing environment while still maximizing yield. The sustainable approach to pest management in radish microgreens cultivation supports both the health of the plants and the well-being of the consumers.

Lastly, the health benefits of incorporating radish microgreens into your diet extend beyond basic nutrition. They are known to support digestion, enhance liver function, and even boost immune responses. The presence of glucosinolates, compounds found in radishes, has been linked to cancer prevention, making these microgreens a powerful ally in maintaining overall health. Embracing radish microgreens not only enriches your meals but also contributes significantly to your wellness journey. By integrating these tiny greens into your lifestyle, you take a proactive step toward achieving a healthier, more vibrant life.

Chapter 2: Nutritional Benefits of Radish Microgreens

Packed with Nutrients

Radish microgreens are a powerhouse of nutrients that can significantly enhance any health-conscious individual's diet. These tiny greens, packed with vitamins and minerals, offer an impressive nutritional profile that rivals many of the more traditional vegetables we often rely on. Just a small handful of radish microgreens can provide a substantial boost of essential nutrients, making them an ideal choice for those looking to improve their overall health and wellbeing. From vitamin C to a wealth of antioxidants, these microgreens deliver a concentrated dose of goodness that can support your immune system and promote overall vitality.

One of the most remarkable aspects of radish microgreens is their high concentration of vitamin C, which is crucial for maintaining healthy skin and a robust immune system. This vitamin helps in the production of collagen, essential for skin elasticity and wound healing. Additionally, radish microgreens contain significant amounts of vitamin K, which plays a vital role in bone health and aids in blood clotting. Including these nutrient-dense greens in your meals can be a simple yet effective way to enhance your nutrient intake without overhauling your entire diet.

In addition to vitamins, radish microgreens are also rich in essential minerals such as magnesium, potassium, and calcium. Magnesium supports muscle and nerve function, while potassium helps regulate blood pressure and fluid balance in the body. Calcium is well-known for its role in maintaining strong bones and teeth. By incorporating radish microgreens into your meals, you can ensure you're getting a variety of essential nutrients that contribute to your body's overall functionality.

Moreover, the antioxidants found in radish microgreens, including glucosinolates, have been shown to have cancer-fighting properties. These compounds help neutralize harmful free radicals in the body, which can lead to chronic diseases. By integrating radish microgreens into your diet, you not only enjoy their vibrant flavors but also take proactive steps toward maintaining your health and reducing the risk of disease. This makes them an excellent addition to salads, sandwiches, and smoothies, effectively enhancing both taste and nutrition.

For those engaged in urban farming or interested in sustainable practices, cultivating radish microgreens is a rewarding endeavor. They require minimal space and can be grown indoors or outdoors, making them ideal for urban environments. By growing your own radish microgreens, you can ensure that they are organic and free from harmful pesticides, all while enjoying the satisfaction of nurturing your own food. This sustainable approach not only benefits your health but also contributes to a more environmentally friendly lifestyle, allowing you to enjoy the big benefits of tiny greens.

Antioxidants and Their Role in Health

Antioxidants play a crucial role in maintaining our health, and their presence in our diet can significantly enhance our overall well-being. These powerful compounds are found in various foods, including radish microgreens, and are known for their ability to neutralize harmful free radicals in the body. By combating oxidative stress, antioxidants help prevent cellular damage, reduce inflammation, and lower the risk of chronic diseases. Incorporating radish microgreens into your meals can be an effortless way to boost your antioxidant intake while enjoying their vibrant flavor and crisp texture.

Radish microgreens are particularly rich in vitamins A, C, and E, all of which are potent antioxidants. Vitamin C, for example, not only supports immune function but also promotes skin health and helps the body absorb iron from plant-based foods. Meanwhile, vitamin E is vital for protecting cell membranes and has been linked to reduced risks of heart disease. By cultivating and consuming organic radish microgreens, you can enjoy these health benefits while supporting sustainable farming practices and enhancing your culinary dishes.

For health-conscious individuals, understanding the importance of antioxidants is essential for making informed dietary choices. By incorporating radish microgreens into your diet, you can easily increase your intake of these vital nutrients. Whether sprinkled on salads, blended into smoothies, or used as a garnish for various dishes, radish microgreens provide a flavorful and nutritious addition that packs a powerful health punch. Embracing these microgreens can be an enjoyable way to ensure you're getting the antioxidants your body needs to thrive.

Urban farming initiatives have made it easier than ever to grow your own radish microgreens at home, even in the smallest of spaces. This accessibility allows you to take control of your food sources and cultivate a diverse array of nutrient-rich crops. By engaging in urban farming, you not only reap the health benefits of antioxidants from radish microgreens but also contribute to a more sustainable food system. The satisfaction of watching your microgreens grow and then incorporating them into your meals can be a rewarding experience for anyone looking to enhance their health.

Incorporating radish microgreens into your daily meals is a delicious way to prioritize your health and well-being. By choosing these tiny greens, you are making a conscious decision to nourish your body with antioxidants that fight free radicals and promote overall health. As you explore the culinary possibilities of radish microgreens, remember that each bite is a step towards a healthier lifestyle, one that embraces the power of nature and the benefits of sustainable practices. Your journey towards well-being starts with these small yet impactful greens, offering big benefits for your health.

Supporting Digestive Health

Supporting digestive health is crucial for overall well-being, and incorporating radish microgreens into your diet can play a significant role in this. Packed with essential nutrients, these tiny greens are not only flavorful but also contribute positively to gut health. Rich in fiber, radish microgreens help promote healthy digestion by facilitating the movement of food through the digestive tract. This can prevent issues such as constipation and bloating, making them an excellent addition to your meals.

In addition to their fiber content, radish microgreens contain a wealth of vitamins and minerals that support digestive function. They are particularly high in vitamin C, which has been shown to enhance the absorption of iron from plant-based foods, further promoting a healthy digestive environment. The presence of antioxidants in radish microgreens also aids in reducing inflammation in the gut, fostering a balanced microbiome. By nourishing your body with these greens, you are investing in long-term digestive health.

For those who are health-conscious and interested in urban farming, growing your own radish microgreens is an empowering practice. It not only ensures a fresh supply of nutrients but also allows you to engage in a sustainable lifestyle. With minimal space and resources, you can cultivate these microgreens at home, knowing that you are producing food that contributes positively to your health. This hands-on approach to food production can enhance your appreciation for what you eat and its impact on your body.

In the kitchen, radish microgreens can be creatively incorporated into a variety of dishes, adding both flavor and nutritional value. Their peppery taste makes them a delightful addition to salads, sandwiches, and wraps. By replacing traditional greens with radish microgreens, you can elevate your meals while reaping their digestive benefits. Experimenting with these microgreens can inspire you to explore new recipes and flavors, making healthy eating an enjoyable experience.

As you embrace the benefits of radish microgreens, remember that supporting your digestive health is a journey. By making small changes, such as incorporating these microgreens into your daily diet, you can foster a healthier gut and overall well-being. The commitment to a nutritious lifestyle, coupled with sustainable farming practices, not only benefits your health but also contributes to a healthier planet. Celebrate the power of radish microgreens, and let them be a vibrant part of your path to wellness.

Chapter 3: Cultivating Organic Radish Microgreens

Choosing the Right Seeds

Choosing the right seeds is a crucial step in cultivating radish microgreens that not only thrive but also deliver the maximum nutritional benefits. When selecting seeds, look for organic options that are specifically labeled for microgreen production. These seeds have been cultivated to ensure high germination rates and superior flavor profiles, which are essential for both health benefits and culinary uses. Many health-conscious individuals prioritize organic seeds, as they are free from harmful pesticides and chemicals, making them a safer choice for your home garden.

Consider the variety of radish seeds available to you. Different types of radish microgreens can yield distinct flavors and textures. For instance, Daikon radish seeds produce a peppery microgreen that can enhance the taste of salads and sandwiches, while the more mild variety, such as Red Globe, offers a subtle crunch. Exploring these varieties not only adds diversity to your meals but also allows you to customize your microgreen garden to suit your palate and nutritional needs.

Make sure to source your seeds from reputable suppliers who prioritize quality and sustainability. Many local nurseries and online retailers specialize in organic microgreen seeds. By supporting these businesses, you contribute to a more sustainable farming ecosystem and ensure that your microgreens are grown from seeds that have been handled with care. Reading reviews and seeking recommendations can help you find the best sources for high-quality seeds, which is essential for a successful growing experience.

As you prepare to plant your seeds, consider the environmental conditions of your growing space. Radish microgreens thrive in well-drained soil and require adequate light, so choosing seeds that are suited to your specific environment is vital. Some varieties may perform better in low-light conditions, while others might need more sunlight to reach their full potential. Pay attention to the growing instructions provided by the seed supplier to ensure optimal growth and maximize the benefits of your microgreens.

Finally, cultivating radish microgreens from carefully chosen seeds is not just about growing food; it's also about embracing a lifestyle centered on health and wellness. By investing time in selecting the right seeds, you are committing to a sustainable practice that nourishes both your body and the planet. The joy of harvesting your own radish microgreens and incorporating them into your meals will not only enhance your culinary creations but also empower you to make healthier choices for yourself and your family. With each seed planted, you are taking a step towards better health and a more sustainable future.

Soil and Growing Medium Options

When embarking on the rewarding journey of growing radish microgreens, selecting the right soil or growing medium is paramount to ensuring vibrant and nutrient-rich crops. For health-conscious individuals, the choice of substrate not only influences the growth rate and flavor of the microgreens but also impacts their nutritional value. A well-balanced growing medium will provide essential nutrients, retain moisture, and allow for proper drainage, creating the ideal environment for these tiny greens to flourish.

Organic potting soil is a popular choice among urban farmers and microgreen enthusiasts alike. This medium typically contains compost, peat moss, and perlite, providing an excellent balance of aeration and moisture retention. By opting for organic, you can ensure that no harmful chemicals are introduced into your microgreens, aligning perfectly with your health-conscious lifestyle. Additionally, organic potting soil is rich in beneficial microorganisms that can enhance plant growth and bolster nutritional content, making it an ideal choice for cultivating radish microgreens.

Alternatively, soilless growing mediums such as coconut coir or hydroponic mats offer unique advantages. Coconut coir, derived from the fibrous husk of coconuts, is an eco-friendly option that provides excellent drainage and aeration. It is also sustainable and renewable, making it a favorite for those committed to environmentally friendly practices. Hydroponic mats, on the other hand, allow for efficient water and nutrient absorption while minimizing the risk of soil-borne diseases. Both options can lead to healthier, more robust radish microgreens while ensuring that your growing practices remain sustainable.

In addition to traditional growing mediums, experimenting with homemade mixes can yield impressive results. Combining ingredients like vermiculite, perlite, and organic compost can create a customized blend that meets the specific needs of your radish microgreens. This approach not only allows for greater control over nutrient levels but also fosters a deeper connection to the growing process. As you cultivate your own blends, you can discover the perfect combination that promotes the growth of nutritious and flavorful microgreens tailored to your taste.

Ultimately, the choice of soil or growing medium directly impacts the success of your radish microgreens. By selecting high-quality, organic, and sustainable options, you are setting the stage for a bountiful harvest that not only supports your health goals but also contributes positively to the environment. Embrace the journey of growing these microgreens, knowing that the choices you make in your growing mediums will lead to vibrant, delicious, and nutrient-packed results that can enhance both your culinary creations and your overall well-being.

Light and Water Requirements

When cultivating radish microgreens, understanding their light and water requirements is essential for achieving a vibrant and nutritious crop. These tiny greens thrive in bright, indirect sunlight, making them perfect for urban farming environments where space might be limited. Ideally, they need around 12 to 16 hours of light each day to grow strong and healthy. If natural sunlight is insufficient, consider using grow lights that provide the full spectrum of light. This approach not only ensures optimal growth but also enhances the nutritional profile of the microgreens, aligning perfectly with your health-conscious lifestyle.

Water is another critical component in the successful cultivation of radish microgreens. These greens prefer a consistently moist environment, but it's important to strike the right balance. Overwatering can lead to root rot, while underwatering can cause the delicate greens to wilt. A well-draining soil mix coupled with a gentle watering method, such as a spray bottle or a watering can with a fine spout, will help maintain the necessary moisture levels. By paying close attention to your watering schedule, you can foster an environment that promotes healthy growth and maximizes the nutritional benefits of your microgreens.

For those who are new to microgreens farming, it may be beneficial to invest in moisture-retaining growing mediums, such as coconut coir or peat moss. These materials not only help retain moisture but also provide the right aeration for the roots to thrive. Regularly checking the moisture level of your growing medium is a simple yet effective practice that can enhance your cultivation experience. Remember, the goal is to create a nurturing environment where your radish microgreens can flourish, delivering their impressive health benefits straight to your plate.

In addition to proper light and water management, consider your growing environment carefully. Radish microgreens prefer temperatures between 60°F and 75°F, which supports both their growth rate and flavor development. By keeping your indoor farming area at a comfortable temperature and ensuring adequate air circulation, you can further promote healthy growth. This attention to detail not only yields a better crop but also contributes to a sustainable practice, as healthy plants are more resilient to pests and diseases.

Ultimately, cultivating radish microgreens with optimal light and water conditions is a rewarding experience that pays off in both flavor and nutrition. These tiny powerhouses are not just easy to grow; they're also packed with vitamins, minerals, and antioxidants that can enhance your overall health and wellness. As you embark on this journey of urban farming and sustainable practices, remember that every small step you take contributes to a larger movement towards healthier living and greater awareness of the food we consume. Embrace the process, enjoy the journey, and relish the benefits of your homegrown radish microgreens.

Chapter 4: Radish Microgreens for Urban Farming

Urban Farming: An Overview

Urban farming has emerged as a revolutionary approach to food production, particularly in densely populated areas where access to fresh produce can be limited. As cities grow and people become more health-conscious, the demand for locally sourced, nutrient-rich food has never been higher. Urban farming not only addresses this need but also empowers individuals to connect with their food sources, making it possible to cultivate fresh ingredients right at home. Among the various options available, growing radish microgreens stands out as a particularly rewarding endeavor that combines ease of cultivation with impressive health benefits.

Radish microgreens are packed with essential nutrients, offering a concentrated source of vitamins and minerals that can enhance any diet. These tiny greens contain high levels of vitamins A, C, E, and K, along with vital antioxidants and fiber. Their nutritional profile makes them an excellent choice for health-conscious individuals looking to boost their wellness routines. Moreover, the quick growth cycle of radish microgreens—typically ready for harvest in just 7 to 14 days—makes them an ideal crop for urban farming, allowing anyone to enjoy the fruits of their labor in a matter of weeks.

The cultivation of radish microgreens in urban settings promotes sustainable farming practices that can significantly reduce the carbon footprint associated with food production. By growing these greens locally, urban farmers can minimize the need for transportation, packaging, and refrigeration, which are often required for store-bought produce. This localized approach not only fosters a sense of community among urban dwellers but also encourages responsible consumption and environmental stewardship. Simple techniques such as using organic soil and natural pest management strategies ensure that the cultivation process remains eco-friendly, further enhancing the appeal of urban farming.

In addition to their health benefits and sustainability, radish microgreens serve as a versatile culinary ingredient that can elevate any dish. Their peppery flavor adds a delightful kick to salads, sandwiches, and smoothies, making them an appealing addition for those seeking to incorporate more greens into their diets. Experimenting with radish microgreens in the kitchen can inspire creativity, encouraging health-conscious individuals to explore new recipes and cooking techniques. By making these vibrant greens a staple in everyday meals, urban farmers can significantly contribute to a healthier lifestyle.

Urban farming, particularly through the cultivation of radish microgreens, presents an exciting opportunity for anyone looking to embrace a healthier, more sustainable way of living. By taking advantage of available space and resources, individuals can grow their own nutrient-dense food while enjoying the therapeutic benefits of gardening. The journey into urban farming not only yields a bountiful harvest but also fosters a deeper appreciation for the food we consume and the environment we inhabit. With each tiny green harvested, urban farmers are not just growing food; they are cultivating health, community, and a brighter future.

Setting Up Your Urban Farm

Setting up your urban farm is an exciting journey that can transform not only your living space but also your lifestyle. By cultivating radish microgreens, you can create a sustainable and nutritious food source right in your own home. The beauty of urban farming is that it allows you to utilize limited space creatively, whether you have a small balcony, a rooftop, or even a windowsill. With a little planning and the right tools, you can grow your own vibrant microgreens, adding a burst of flavor and nutrition to your meals while contributing positively to your health and wellness.

To begin, it's essential to choose the right location for your urban farm. Look for a spot that receives ample sunlight, ideally six to eight hours a day, which is crucial for the growth of radish microgreens. If natural light is limited, consider investing in grow lights to provide the necessary illumination. Ensure that your chosen area has good air circulation to prevent mold and other issues. The beauty of microgreens is that they can thrive in small containers, so feel free to get creative with recycled materials like food containers or shallow trays. This not only saves money but also promotes sustainable practices, which are at the heart of urban farming.

Next, gather the supplies you'll need to kickstart your microgreen adventure. You will need high-quality organic radish seeds, potting soil, and containers for planting. Organic seeds ensure that you are growing your microgreens without harmful chemicals, which aligns perfectly with a health-conscious lifestyle. Choose a soil that provides good drainage and is rich in nutrients. As you set up your containers, remember to sow the seeds densely, as radish microgreens grow quickly and can be harvested within a week to ten days. This fast turnaround makes them an excellent choice for urban farmers looking to enjoy the fruits of their labor in no time.

Pest management is another critical aspect of setting up your urban farm. While radish microgreens are relatively resistant to pests, it's important to keep your growing environment clean and monitor for any signs of trouble. Implementing preventive measures, such as maintaining good airflow and avoiding overwatering, can significantly reduce the risk of pests. If you do encounter any issues, consider using organic pest management solutions, such as neem oil or insecticidal soap, to keep your microgreens healthy without compromising your commitment to organic practices. Your proactive approach to pest management will ensure that your urban farm remains a thriving oasis of health.

Finally, don't forget to enjoy the culinary benefits of your radish microgreens. These tiny greens pack a punch of flavor and can elevate any dish, from salads to sandwiches, and even soups. Incorporating them into your meals not only enhances taste but also boosts nutritional value, as radish microgreens are rich in vitamins and antioxidants. As you harvest your microgreens, take a moment to appreciate the journey you've embarked on. You are not just growing food; you are cultivating a lifestyle that prioritizes health, sustainability, and self-sufficiency. Embrace this rewarding endeavor, and let your urban farm flourish!

Maximizing Small Spaces

Maximizing small spaces for growing radish microgreens is not only a practical approach for urban dwellers but also a rewarding endeavor that can yield significant health benefits. Whether you have a tiny balcony, a windowsill, or just a small corner in your home, you can create an efficient microgreen garden that thrives in limited conditions. By understanding the essentials of microgreen cultivation and making the most of your available area, you can enjoy fresh, nutritious radish microgreens year-round.

Vertical gardening techniques can significantly enhance your ability to grow microgreens in small spaces. Using shelves, wall-mounted planters, or even repurposed furniture, you can create a multi-layered growing area. This method allows you to increase your yield without requiring more horizontal space. Furthermore, incorporating hydroponic systems can help you maximize water efficiency and nutrient delivery, ensuring your radish microgreens flourish even in compact environments.

Choosing the right containers is crucial to optimizing your small gardening area. Look for shallow trays that provide ample drainage while maximizing surface area. These trays can be stacked or placed side by side to utilize every inch of your space. When selecting potting media, consider lightweight options that retain moisture and nutrients, such as coconut coir or seed-starting mixes. This choice not only supports healthy growth but also simplifies maintenance, allowing you to focus on enjoying your fresh greens.

Lighting is another vital factor in maximizing your small space. If natural sunlight is limited, consider using LED grow lights, which are energy-efficient and can be positioned directly above your microgreens. These lights can mimic the sun's spectrum, promoting vigorous growth even in poorly lit areas. By managing your light exposure and ensuring your radish microgreens receive adequate illumination, you can optimize their growth potential and enhance their nutritional benefits.

Incorporating sustainable practices in your small-space microgreens garden is not only beneficial for your health but also for the environment. Utilizing organic seeds and pest management techniques such as companion planting or natural deterrents can help maintain a healthy growing environment. By committing to sustainable methods, you contribute to a healthier planet while enjoying the delicious and nutritious rewards of your radish microgreens. Embrace the journey of microgreen gardening, and discover how even the smallest spaces can lead to big benefits for your health and well-being.

Chapter 5: Pest Management in Radish Microgreens Production

Common Pests and How to Identify Them

When cultivating radish microgreens, it's essential to be aware of common pests that may threaten your delicate plants. Identifying these pests early on can make a significant difference in the health of your crop and ultimately your well-being. Pests like aphids, whiteflies, and spider mites can invade your microgreen trays, but with a little knowledge, you can spot them before they wreak havoc on your greens.

Aphids are small, soft-bodied insects that often cluster on the undersides of leaves. They come in various colors, including green, black, and yellow. You can identify them by their pear-shaped bodies and their tendency to leave a sticky residue known as honeydew, which can attract other pests and lead to fungal diseases. Keeping an eye out for these tiny invaders is crucial, as they reproduce quickly and can cause significant damage in a short amount of time.

Whiteflies are another common pest that microgreen growers may encounter. These tiny, white, moth-like insects tend to fly up in a cloud when disturbed. They prefer warm conditions and are often found on the undersides of leaves, feeding on the sap of your microgreens. If you notice yellowing leaves or a sticky film on the surface of your growing medium, it may be time to investigate for whiteflies. Early detection can help you implement effective management strategies before they become a serious problem.

Spider mites, although not true insects, are also a threat to radish microgreens. These minute arachnids are often identified by the fine webbing they create on the plants and the speckled appearance they leave on leaves due to their feeding habits. If you see tiny dots or discoloration on your microgreens, inspect closely for spider mites. Their presence can lead to weakened plants and diminished nutrient quality, so prompt action is essential for maintaining a healthy crop.

Understanding how to identify these common pests is a crucial step in sustainable radish microgreens farming. By being vigilant and proactive in your approach, you can protect your plants while minimizing the need for chemical interventions. Embracing organic pest management strategies not only ensures the vitality of your microgreens but also reinforces your commitment to health and wellness through clean, nutritious food. Celebrate the journey of urban farming, knowing that each step you take leads to a more sustainable and health-conscious lifestyle.

Organic Pest Control Methods

Organic pest control methods are essential for maintaining the health of radish microgreens while ensuring that the cultivation process aligns with your values of sustainability and wellness. As health-conscious individuals, you understand that what you consume should be free from harmful chemicals. By adopting organic pest control strategies, you can cultivate vibrant, nutritious radish microgreens that not only nourish your body but also contribute positively to the environment.

One effective approach to organic pest control is the use of beneficial insects. Ladybugs, lacewings, and predatory mites are natural allies in the fight against pests that may threaten your microgreens. These insects target common pests such as aphids and spider mites, allowing your radish microgreens to thrive without the need for synthetic pesticides. By creating a welcoming environment for these beneficial species, you can promote a balanced ecosystem in your urban farming setup, enhancing both plant health and biodiversity.

Another method worth considering is the application of natural repellents. Essential oils derived from plants like neem, peppermint, and rosemary can deter unwanted pests while being gentle on your microgreens. These natural solutions not only protect your crops but also align with the ethos of organic farming. Incorporating these oils into your pest management routine can provide peace of mind as you nurture your radish microgreens, knowing you are doing so without compromising their safety or your health.

Companion planting is another organic technique that can greatly benefit your radish microgreens. By planting certain herbs and flowers alongside your microgreens, you can naturally repel pests and attract beneficial insects. For instance, planting marigolds can deter nematodes, while basil can help ward off aphids. This method not only enhances pest management but also creates a diverse and visually appealing garden space, reinforcing the connection between healthy plants and a healthy lifestyle.

Finally, maintaining proper sanitation and cultural practices is crucial in organic pest control. Regularly cleaning your growing area, rotating crops, and ensuring adequate air circulation can significantly reduce pest populations. By fostering an environment that prioritizes cleanliness and plant health, you'll set the stage for successful radish microgreens cultivation. Embracing these organic pest control methods ensures that your journey into growing radish microgreens remains fruitful, enjoyable, and aligned with your commitment to health and sustainability.

Preventive Measures for Healthy Crops

Preventive measures are essential for ensuring the health and vitality of radish microgreens. By adopting a proactive approach to cultivation, health-conscious individuals can maximize not only the yield but also the nutritional benefits of these tiny greens. The first step in this journey involves understanding the importance of soil health. Using organic soil amendments like compost and aged manure enriches the soil with essential nutrients, promoting a robust foundation for growth. This not only enhances the flavor of the microgreens but also ensures they are packed with vitamins, minerals, and antioxidants that contribute to overall wellness.

Water management is another crucial aspect of preventive measures. Radish microgreens thrive in a well-balanced environment, which means that both overwatering and underwatering can lead to poor growth and increased susceptibility to diseases. Implementing a consistent watering schedule along with using a moisture meter can help maintain optimal conditions. Additionally, employing techniques such as bottom watering can prevent issues related to damping-off, a common fungal disease that affects seedlings. By taking these steps, cultivators can foster a healthy environment that encourages vigorous growth while minimizing health risks to the crops.

Pest management plays a vital role in the cultivation of radish microgreens, especially in urban farming settings where space is limited. Integrating natural pest deterrents, such as companion planting with herbs like basil or cilantro, can create a balanced ecosystem that naturally repels harmful insects. Regular monitoring for signs of pests and diseases enables growers to act swiftly, ensuring that any issues are addressed before they escalate. Utilizing organic pest control methods, such as insecticidal soap or neem oil, further supports the health of the microgreens while aligning with sustainable practices that health-conscious consumers value.

Maintaining proper air circulation is another preventive measure that cannot be overlooked.

Crowded environments can lead to increased humidity levels, creating a breeding ground for molds and mildew. By spacing the trays appropriately and using fans to promote airflow, cultivators can create an ideal setting for their radish microgreens to thrive. This not only contributes to the health of the crops but also enhances the flavor and nutritional profile of the microgreens, making them an even more appealing addition to a healthy diet.

Finally, education and continuous learning are key preventive measures that empower growers to cultivate healthy radish microgreens effectively. Engaging with community workshops, online resources, and local gardening groups allows individuals to stay informed about the best practices and innovations in microgreens cultivation. Sharing experiences and learning from others can lead to new ideas and techniques that promote sustainability and health. By embracing a culture of knowledge and collaboration, health-conscious individuals can inspire one another to grow not only nutritious microgreens but also a thriving community of sustainable practices.

Chapter 6: Culinary Uses of Radish Microgreens

Adding Flavor and Texture to Dishes

Radish microgreens are a powerhouse of flavor and texture that can transform your dishes into vibrant culinary experiences. These tiny greens pack a peppery punch that can elevate even the simplest of meals. Whether you're garnishing a salad, adding depth to a sandwich, or enhancing a stir-fry, the distinct taste of radish microgreens brings an exciting dimension to your cooking. Their bold flavor not only excites the palate but also complements a wide range of ingredients, making them versatile additions to both everyday meals and gourmet creations.

In addition to their remarkable flavor, radish microgreens provide a delightful crunch that can enhance the overall texture of a dish. Their tender yet crisp leaves contrast beautifully with softer components, such as creamy dressings or tender proteins. This textural interplay not only makes your meals more enjoyable but also encourages mindful eating. The act of savoring each bite becomes a sensory experience, allowing you to appreciate the nuances of flavor and texture that these microgreens offer.

Incorporating radish microgreens into your cooking is not only a culinary adventure but also a commitment to health and wellness. Rich in vitamins, minerals, and antioxidants, these microgreens can contribute significantly to your daily nutritional intake. By adding them to your meals, you are not only enhancing flavor and texture but also boosting the overall health benefits of your dishes. This makes them an ideal choice for health-conscious individuals looking to nourish their bodies while enjoying vibrant flavors.

Urban farming has made it easier than ever to grow your own radish microgreens, allowing you to embrace sustainable practices in your culinary endeavors. With a little effort, you can cultivate these nutrient-dense greens right in your kitchen or balcony, ensuring that you're using the freshest ingredients possible. This connection to your food source fosters a sense of empowerment and responsibility, encouraging you to explore new recipes and cooking techniques that highlight the unique qualities of radish microgreens.

Finally, the culinary possibilities with radish microgreens are endless. From enhancing the flavor of soups and stews to adding a fresh touch to tacos and wraps, the creativity you can unleash is limited only by your imagination. Experimenting with different pairings and presentation styles will not only impress your guests but also inspire you to make healthy eating a delightful and enjoyable part of your lifestyle. Embrace the power of radish microgreens, and watch as they transform your dishes into vibrant celebrations of flavor and health.

Creative Recipes Featuring Radish Microgreens

Radish microgreens are not only a nutritional powerhouse but also a vibrant addition to your culinary repertoire. Their peppery flavor and crisp texture make them an ideal ingredient for a variety of dishes. Incorporating radish microgreens into your meals is a delightful way to boost both flavor and health benefits. Whether you are looking to enhance salads, sandwiches, or even main dishes, these tiny greens can elevate your cooking while providing a plethora of vitamins, minerals, and antioxidants that support overall wellness.

One creative way to enjoy radish microgreens is by adding them to your morning smoothie. Simply toss a handful into your blender along with your favorite fruits, a banana for creaminess, and a splash of almond milk. The microgreens will blend seamlessly, adding a subtle peppery note and a vibrant green hue to your drink. This invigorating smoothie not only tastes great but also delivers a concentrated dose of nutrients to kick-start your day, making it a perfect choice for health-conscious individuals.

For lunch or dinner, consider crafting a refreshing radish microgreen salad. Start with a base of mixed greens, then layer on sliced cucumbers, cherry tomatoes, and avocado. Top it off with a generous handful of radish microgreens for that extra crunch and zing. Drizzle with a simple dressing of olive oil, lemon juice, salt, and pepper to allow the microgreens' flavor to shine through. This salad is not only visually appealing but also packed with essential nutrients, making it a satisfying and healthful meal option.

Radish microgreens can also be a fantastic addition to gourmet sandwiches or wraps. Spread a layer of hummus or avocado on whole-grain bread or a tortilla, then pile on your favorite veggies, protein, and a good serving of radish microgreens. The peppery taste of the microgreens complements the other ingredients beautifully, adding both texture and a pop of flavor. This makes for a quick, nutritious lunch that aligns with sustainable eating practices, especially when you source your ingredients from local farms or grow your own microgreens at home.

Lastly, elevate your culinary creations by incorporating radish microgreens into your cooking as a finishing touch. Sprinkle them atop roasted vegetables, grain bowls, or even pizza for an extra boost of flavor and nutrition. Their vibrant color and unique taste can transform any dish into a gourmet experience while adding essential vitamins and minerals. Embracing radish microgreens in your kitchen not only enhances your meals but also supports a healthy lifestyle and sustainable food practices, making them a must-have ingredient for the health-conscious cook.

Incorporating Microgreens into Everyday Meals

Incorporating microgreens into everyday meals is an effortless way to enhance both flavor and nutrition. Radish microgreens, in particular, are a powerhouse of vitamins and minerals, making them an ideal choice for health-conscious individuals looking to elevate their culinary creations. These tiny greens can easily be added to salads, sandwiches, smoothies, and even soups, providing a peppery kick that enlivens any dish. By integrating radish microgreens into your meals, you not only boost their nutritional content but also support vibrant flavors that can transform simple recipes into gourmet experiences.

One of the simplest ways to enjoy radish microgreens is by tossing them into salads. Their crisp texture and bold flavor complement a variety of ingredients, from mixed greens to fresh vegetables. Try layering them on top of a bed of arugula, cucumbers, and cherry tomatoes, drizzled with a light vinaigrette. This not only adds a delightful crunch but also infuses your salad with vitamins A, C, and K, along with essential minerals. For those who enjoy meal prep, consider batch-making salads with radish microgreens as a staple ingredient. This way, you can ensure that every bite is packed with nutrients.

Radish microgreens also shine in sandwiches and wraps, where they can replace traditional lettuce. Their robust flavor pairs well with meats, cheeses, and spreads, making them a perfect addition to a turkey or hummus wrap. By choosing radish microgreens, you add a unique twist to your lunch while reaping the benefits of their high antioxidant content. Even simple snacks, such as avocado toast, can be elevated with a sprinkle of these greens, turning an ordinary meal into a healthful delight.

For those who enjoy smoothies, incorporating radish microgreens can be both nutritious and refreshing. Blend a handful of these greens with fruits like bananas, apples, or berries, and add a splash of almond milk for a vibrant, nutrient-packed drink. The peppery notes of radish microgreens can provide a surprising depth of flavor, making your smoothie not only a health booster but also a culinary adventure. This is an excellent way to start your day or refuel after a workout, ensuring you meet your daily vegetable intake with ease.

Finally, consider using radish microgreens as a garnish for soups and stews. Their bright green color adds visual appeal, while their flavor enhances the overall dish. A sprinkle of these microgreens on top of creamy potato soup or spicy chili can elevate the presentation and taste, inviting you to explore new culinary horizons. By making radish microgreens a regular component of your meals, you are not just feeding your body; you are embracing sustainable practices and supporting your health and wellness journey in a delicious way.

Chapter 7: Sustainable Practices in Radish Microgreens Farming

The Importance of Sustainability

The importance of sustainability in our food systems cannot be overstated, especially when it comes to the cultivation of radish microgreens. As health-conscious individuals, embracing sustainable practices not only benefits our personal health but also contributes positively to the planet. By prioritizing sustainability in microgreens farming, we can ensure that our food sources are not only nutritious but also environmentally friendly. This holistic approach aligns our dietary choices with our values, promoting a healthier lifestyle while safeguarding the earth for future generations.

Sustainable practices in radish microgreens cultivation involve a careful selection of organic methods that minimize environmental impact. By using organic seeds and natural fertilizers, we can promote soil health and biodiversity. This is particularly important in urban farming, where space is limited and the need for efficient, eco-friendly practices is crucial. Urban dwellers can easily incorporate radish microgreens into their diets by growing them in small spaces, thereby reducing their carbon footprint and fostering a connection to their food sources.

Beyond environmental considerations, the nutritional benefits of radish microgreens make them a powerhouse addition to any diet. Packed with vitamins, minerals, and antioxidants, these tiny greens provide a significant health boost in a small package. By choosing sustainably grown radish microgreens, we are not only nourishing our bodies but also supporting agricultural practices that prioritize health and wellness. This conscious choice can inspire a ripple effect, encouraging others to adopt similar habits and contribute to a more sustainable future.

Pest management is another crucial aspect of sustainable radish microgreens farming. By utilizing integrated pest management techniques, farmers can protect their crops without resorting to harmful chemicals. This approach not only ensures that the microgreens remain healthy and safe to eat but also promotes a balanced ecosystem. When consumers prioritize sustainably produced radish microgreens, they are supporting farming methods that respect nature and promote biodiversity, which is essential for long-term agricultural success.

Incorporating radish microgreens into culinary creations not only enhances flavor but also underscores the importance of sustainability in our food choices. Chefs and home cooks alike can elevate their dishes with these vibrant greens while also making a statement about their commitment to health and sustainability. By championing the use of radish microgreens, we can inspire others to explore the benefits of sustainable eating and foster a greater appreciation for the interconnectedness of our health, our food, and our planet. Together, we can cultivate a future where sustainability is at the heart of our food choices, creating a lasting impact on our health and the environment.

Eco-Friendly Growing Techniques

Eco-friendly growing techniques are essential for cultivating radish microgreens that are not only nutritious but also sustainable. By adopting these practices, health-conscious individuals can enjoy the benefits of fresh, organic produce while minimizing their ecological footprint. Embracing eco-friendly methods allows urban farmers to create green spaces that contribute positively to their local environments, making it a win-win situation for both growers and consumers.

One of the most effective eco-friendly techniques is utilizing organic growing mediums. Organic soil alternatives, such as coconut coir, compost, and peat moss, enrich the growing environment without harmful chemicals. These materials improve soil structure and retain moisture, promoting healthy root development in radish microgreens. By choosing organic mediums, growers ensure that their microgreens are free from synthetic fertilizers, which can leach into waterways and disrupt local ecosystems.

Water conservation is another vital aspect of eco-friendly growing techniques. Implementing drip irrigation systems or using self-watering containers can significantly reduce water consumption while providing consistent hydration for radish microgreens. Additionally, capturing rainwater for irrigation not only conserves resources but also enhances the nutrient profile of the microgreens, as rainwater is often naturally softer and free from chlorine. This approach not only benefits the microgreens but also contributes to a sustainable urban farming practice.

Pest management is crucial for maintaining an eco-friendly growing environment. Instead of relying on chemical pesticides, growers can utilize natural pest deterrents such as neem oil or insecticidal soap. Furthermore, encouraging beneficial insects, like ladybugs and lacewings, can help control pest populations naturally. By fostering a balanced ecosystem, urban farmers can protect their radish microgreens while promoting biodiversity, which is essential for a healthy environment.

Lastly, practicing crop rotation and companion planting can enhance the sustainability of radish microgreens cultivation. By rotating crops and planting them alongside compatible species, growers can naturally improve soil health and reduce the risk of pests and diseases. This holistic approach not only supports the growth of vibrant and nutritious microgreens but also contributes to a thriving urban agriculture movement, encouraging individuals to take part in the journey of eco-friendly growing. Embracing these techniques is not just about cultivating food; it's about cultivating a healthier planet for future generations.

Reducing Waste in Microgreens Production

Reducing waste in microgreens production is essential for both the environment and the sustainability of urban farming practices. As health-conscious individuals, it's vital to recognize that every step taken towards minimizing waste contributes to the overall wellbeing of our communities and the planet. By adopting efficient cultivation methods and innovative practices, we can ensure that the benefits of radish microgreens extend beyond their nutritional advantages, promoting a more sustainable food system.

One of the most effective ways to reduce waste is through careful planning and management of resources. This begins with seed selection and usage. By understanding the germination rates and growth cycles of radish microgreens, growers can optimize their seed purchases and reduce excess. Additionally, implementing precise sowing techniques minimizes leftover seeds and maximizes yield. Each seed sown contributes to the potential harvest, ensuring that nothing goes to waste and every nutrient-packed microgreen is utilized.

Another key strategy in waste reduction is the implementation of composting practices. After harvesting, the leftover roots and stems can be composted rather than discarded. This not only reduces the volume of waste sent to landfills but also creates nutrient-rich compost that can enhance future growing cycles. By integrating composting into microgreens production, growers can complete the nutrient cycle and contribute to soil health, which is crucial for sustainable farming.

Water management is also critical in minimizing waste. Efficient irrigation systems, such as drip irrigation or hydroponic methods, can significantly cut down on water usage while ensuring that radish microgreens receive the moisture they need for optimal growth. By closely monitoring water levels and adjusting irrigation schedules based on environmental conditions, producers can avoid overwatering and reduce water waste. This mindful approach not only supports the health of the microgreens but also conserves a precious resource.

Finally, educating consumers about the benefits of radish microgreens and encouraging them to embrace sustainable practices can further reduce waste. By promoting the idea of using every part of the microgreen, from the leaves to the roots, and sharing creative recipes that incorporate radish microgreens, we can inspire a culture of sustainability. When health-conscious individuals choose to support local microgreens producers who prioritize waste reduction, they not only benefit from the nutritional value of these tiny greens but also contribute to a larger movement towards responsible and sustainable food production.

Chapter 8: Radish Microgreens for Health and Wellness

Enhancing Your Diet with Microgreens

Incorporating microgreens into your diet is a simple yet impactful way to enhance your nutritional intake and overall wellness. These tiny greens, particularly radish microgreens, pack a punch when it comes to flavor and health benefits. They are rich in vitamins, minerals, and antioxidants, making them an ideal addition to a health-conscious lifestyle. Whether you're looking to boost your immune system, increase your energy levels, or simply enjoy vibrant flavors, radish microgreens can play a key role in achieving your health goals.

Radish microgreens are incredibly versatile and can be easily integrated into various meals. Their peppery flavor adds a delightful kick to salads, sandwiches, and wraps, while also serving as an eye-catching garnish for soups and entrees. By incorporating these nutrient-dense greens into your meals, you not only enhance the taste but also significantly increase the nutritional profile of your dishes. With their quick growth cycle, you can even cultivate these microgreens at home, ensuring a fresh supply right at your fingertips.

For those interested in sustainable practices, growing radish microgreens is a rewarding venture. They require minimal space and resources, making them perfect for urban farming enthusiasts. With a few simple tools, anyone can start cultivating these microgreens on a windowsill or balcony. This not only contributes to a more sustainable lifestyle by reducing your carbon footprint but also allows you to enjoy the freshest greens possible, harvested just moments before they hit your plate.

In addition to their culinary applications, radish microgreens offer numerous health benefits. They are known to support digestion, promote heart health, and even have anti-inflammatory properties. By incorporating these microgreens into your diet, you can harness their powerful nutrients to bolster your well-being. Regular consumption can contribute to a healthier lifestyle, providing you with the energy and vitality needed to thrive in your daily activities.

Embracing radish microgreens as a staple in your diet is a small change that can lead to significant health improvements. By exploring their culinary potential and understanding their nutritional benefits, you can enhance your meals while nourishing your body. Whether you're a seasoned chef or a kitchen novice, incorporating these tiny greens into your diet is a delightful way to elevate your health and enjoy the many flavors and benefits they bring.

The Role of Radish Microgreens in Detoxification

The role of radish microgreens in detoxification is increasingly recognized among health-conscious individuals seeking natural ways to support their bodies. These tiny greens are not just a culinary delight; they pack a powerful punch when it comes to cleansing the body of harmful toxins. Rich in antioxidants and essential nutrients, radish microgreens contribute to the body's natural detoxification processes, helping to eliminate free radicals and reduce oxidative stress. By incorporating these vibrant greens into your diet, you can enhance your overall well-being while enjoying their crisp, peppery flavor.

Radish microgreens are particularly notable for their high content of glucosinolates, compounds that are known to support liver function. The liver is a crucial organ in the detoxification process, responsible for filtering toxins from the blood and metabolizing substances. The inclusion of radish microgreens in your meals can bolster liver health, promoting efficient detoxification. This makes them an excellent choice for those looking to improve their body's natural ability to cleanse itself, especially in today's environment where exposure to pollutants is commonplace.

In addition to their liver-supporting properties, radish microgreens are also rich in vitamins C and E, both of which play vital roles in maintaining a healthy immune system. A strong immune system is essential for effective detoxification, as it helps the body fight off infections and diseases that can hinder the detox process. By regularly consuming radish microgreens, you can boost your nutrient intake, further enhancing your body's defenses against harmful substances and supporting its ability to detoxify naturally.

Urban farming enthusiasts will find radish microgreens particularly appealing due to their quick growth cycle and minimal space requirements. These greens can be cultivated easily in small environments, making them ideal for city dwellers looking to incorporate fresh produce into their diets. By growing your own radish microgreens, you not only gain access to fresh, nutrient-dense food but also take an active role in your health and wellness journey. This hands-on approach to food production aligns perfectly with sustainable farming practices, allowing individuals to enjoy the benefits of fresh greens while minimizing their ecological footprint.

Incorporating radish microgreens into your daily meals can be a delicious and easy way to enhance your detoxification efforts. Whether sprinkled on salads, blended into smoothies, or used as a garnish for various dishes, these tiny greens offer versatility and flavor. As you embrace the power of radish microgreens, you'll not only nourish your body but also enjoy the process of making healthier choices. Every bite of these vibrant greens can be a step towards a cleaner, healthier lifestyle, reinforcing the idea that small changes can lead to significant benefits for your overall health.

Building a Healthier Lifestyle with Microgreens

In the quest for a healthier lifestyle, incorporating radish microgreens into your diet can be a transformative step. These tiny greens are not only packed with nutrients but also offer a delightful crunch and peppery flavor that can elevate any dish. Adding radish microgreens to your meals is an effortless way to enhance nutritional intake, making it easier to meet your daily requirements for vitamins and minerals. By embracing these vibrant greens, you can create a colorful and healthful plate that supports your wellness goals.

Growing your own radish microgreens is an empowering experience that fosters a deeper connection to your food. Whether you have a spacious garden or a small urban balcony, cultivating these microgreens is accessible to everyone. The process requires minimal space and resources, making it an ideal venture for health-conscious individuals looking to take control of their food source. By engaging in microgreens farming, you can not only enjoy fresher produce but also experience the satisfaction of nurturing plants from seeds to harvest.

The nutritional benefits of radish microgreens are remarkable, as they are rich in essential vitamins such as A, C, and K, and packed with antioxidants. These nutrients play a critical role in supporting overall health, from boosting your immune system to promoting healthy skin. Incorporating radish microgreens into your daily meals can help prevent nutritional deficiencies and encourage a balanced diet. Whether sprinkled on salads, blended into smoothies, or used as a garnish for various dishes, these nutrient-dense greens serve as a flavorful addition that enhances both taste and health.

Sustainable practices in radish microgreens farming also contribute to a healthier lifestyle by promoting environmentally friendly methods. By growing microgreens organically, you reduce your carbon footprint and avoid harmful pesticides that can compromise your health and the planet. Urban farming initiatives are becoming increasingly popular, allowing city dwellers to cultivate their own food and reduce their reliance on store-bought produce. This movement not only supports local ecosystems but also encourages community engagement and awareness around healthy eating practices.

Finally, incorporating radish microgreens into your culinary repertoire is an excellent way to inspire creativity in the kitchen. Their versatility means they can be used in various cuisines, from gourmet dishes to everyday meals. Experimenting with radish microgreens encourages you to explore new flavors and textures, making healthy eating enjoyable and exciting. By prioritizing these tiny greens in your lifestyle, you're not only investing in your health but also embracing a journey of culinary exploration that can lead to lasting wellness.

Chapter 9: Conclusion: Embracing Radish Microgreens

Recap of the Benefits

Radish microgreens represent a remarkable fusion of nutrition and flavor, serving as a powerful addition to a health-conscious diet. Packed with vitamins A, C, E, and K, these tiny greens offer an impressive boost to your immune system. They also contain essential minerals such as calcium, magnesium, and potassium, all of which contribute to overall well-being. For those seeking to enhance their nutritional intake, incorporating radish microgreens into daily meals can be a simple yet effective strategy to increase the essential nutrients that support a healthy lifestyle.

From an environmental perspective, radish microgreens are a sustainable choice for urban farming. Their fast growth cycle, requiring only a couple of weeks from seed to harvest, makes them an ideal crop for small spaces. This quick cultivation not only reduces land requirements but also minimizes water usage compared to traditional farming methods. As urban farming continues to grow in popularity, radish microgreens stand out as a sustainable option that can thrive in limited environments, allowing city dwellers to enjoy nutrient-dense produce right from their homes.

Pest management is a significant concern for any farmer, organic or otherwise. Fortunately, the cultivation of radish microgreens can be integrated into sustainable practices that naturally deter pests. By using methods such as crop rotation, companion planting, and organic pest repellents, growers can maintain healthy microgreen crops without relying on harmful chemicals. This approach not only supports the health of the environment but also ensures that the produce remains safe and nutritious for consumption.

The culinary versatility of radish microgreens is another compelling benefit. Their crisp texture and peppery flavor can elevate a variety of dishes, from salads and sandwiches to soups and smoothies. Adding these microgreens not only enhances the taste but also boosts the aesthetic appeal of meals, making healthy eating more enjoyable. Chefs and home cooks alike can experiment with radish microgreens, discovering new ways to incorporate them into their recipes while reaping the health benefits they offer.

In conclusion, the advantages of radish microgreens extend beyond their nutritional content. Their role in sustainable urban farming, effective pest management, and culinary enhancement makes them a valuable asset in any health-conscious individual's kitchen. Embracing radish microgreens is an empowering choice toward better health, sustainability, and delicious eating. By integrating these tiny greens into your diet, you are not just making a healthy choice for yourself; you are also contributing to a more sustainable future.

Encouragement to Start Growing

Growing your own radish microgreens is an empowering journey that not only enriches your meals but also contributes positively to your health and the environment. The beauty of microgreens lies in their simplicity; they can thrive even in small spaces, making them perfect for anyone, regardless of their living situation. Whether you have a sprawling garden or just a sunny windowsill, starting your own cultivation of radish microgreens is an achievable goal that can bring immense joy and satisfaction. Embrace the opportunity to connect with your food, and take the first steps toward nurturing your own tiny greens.

The nutritional benefits of radish microgreens are remarkable, and incorporating them into your diet can significantly enhance your health. Packed with vitamins, minerals, and antioxidants, these little powerhouses can boost your immune system, improve digestion, and support overall wellness. Imagine the delight of knowing that each bite of your homegrown microgreens is not just delicious but also a gift to your body. By cultivating radish microgreens, you're not just growing a plant; you're nurturing your health and well-being, creating a direct connection between your efforts and the nourishment you receive.

Urban farming is becoming increasingly popular, and radish microgreens are a perfect fit for city dwellers looking to embrace a more sustainable lifestyle. These greens require minimal space and can be grown indoors or outdoors, allowing you to take advantage of limited resources while contributing to local food systems. By starting your own microgreens garden, you're participating in a movement that promotes sustainability and reduces reliance on store-bought produce, which often comes with a hefty environmental cost. Your small efforts can lead to significant positive impacts, both for yourself and your community.

Pest management is a crucial aspect of successful radish microgreens production, but it's easier than you might think. By employing organic methods and focusing on preventive measures, you can cultivate your microgreens without the need for harmful chemicals. Emphasizing sustainable practices not only ensures the purity of your harvest but also fosters a healthy ecosystem around your growing area. This approach supports both the environment and your personal health, allowing you to enjoy fresh, organic microgreens while minimizing your ecological footprint.

As you embark on the adventure of growing radish microgreens, remember that you are not just cultivating plants; you are cultivating a lifestyle centered around health, sustainability, and well-being. This journey will introduce you to new culinary experiences as you experiment with incorporating microgreens into your meals, elevating your dishes with their vibrant flavors and textures. So gather your supplies, find a sunny spot, and start your microgreens garden today. Every small step you take not only benefits you but also contributes to a healthier planet. Your journey towards growing radish microgreens is a chance to celebrate the connection between food, health, and sustainability.

Future Trends in Microgreens Farming

The future of microgreens farming, particularly with radish microgreens, is poised for remarkable growth and innovation. As health-conscious consumers increasingly seek nutrient-dense foods, the demand for microgreens is set to rise significantly. Urban farming is becoming a prominent trend, enabling individuals with limited space to cultivate their own radish microgreens. This movement not only promotes sustainability but also empowers people to take charge of their health by incorporating fresh, organic produce into their diets. As more urban dwellers discover the joy of growing their own food, the landscape of microgreens farming will continue to evolve, making it more accessible to everyone.

Technological advancements are also transforming the microgreens farming sector. Innovations in hydroponics and vertical farming systems allow for year-round cultivation, even in urban environments. These systems can optimize space and resources, making it easier for aspiring farmers to produce high-quality radish microgreens with minimal environmental impact. With the integration of smart farming technologies, such as sensors and automated systems, growers can monitor and manage their crops more efficiently, ensuring optimal growth conditions. This technological shift not only enhances productivity but also attracts a new generation of farmers who are eager to embrace sustainable practices.

Sustainable practices will undoubtedly play a crucial role in the future of radish microgreens farming. As consumers become more aware of the environmental impact of their food choices, there will be an increasing emphasis on organic cultivation methods that reduce chemical inputs and promote biodiversity. Crop rotation, companion planting, and organic pest management will be essential strategies for maintaining healthy soil and productive microgreens. By prioritizing sustainability, farmers can not only grow nutritious greens but also contribute to the health of the planet, fostering a symbiotic relationship between agriculture and the environment.

The culinary potential of radish microgreens is set to gain traction as chefs and home cooks alike recognize their unique flavor and vibrant appearance. As the farm-to-table movement continues to flourish, the incorporation of microgreens into everyday dishes will become more common. This trend opens up exciting opportunities for culinary creativity, encouraging health-conscious individuals to experiment with radish microgreens in salads, sandwiches, and garnishes. With their exceptional nutritional profile, these tiny greens will not only enhance the aesthetic appeal of meals but also provide a powerful boost of vitamins and minerals, making them a staple ingredient in healthy cooking.

Finally, educational initiatives and community engagement will be pivotal in shaping the future of microgreens farming. Workshops, online courses, and social media platforms dedicated to radish microgreens cultivation will empower individuals to learn and share their experiences. As communities come together to promote urban farming, knowledge sharing will encourage more people to take up microgreens farming as a hobby or business. This grassroots movement will foster a stronger connection to food, health, and sustainability, ensuring that the benefits of radish microgreens are accessible to all. Embracing these future trends will not only nourish our bodies but also cultivate a thriving, health-focused community dedicated to well-being and sustainability.

www.ingramcontent.com/pod-product-compliance
Lightning Source LLC
Chambersburg PA
CBHW050811250726
48653CB00006B/2165